How to be Chic in the Winter

Living slim, happy
and stylish during
the cold season

FIONA FERRIS

ISBN-13: 978-1539834960
ISBN-10: 1539834964

CONTENTS

Introduction

Late summer heading into early autumn/fall is such a beautiful time of the year. You can feel everything growing still and soft; nature is slowing down and people are getting cozy. The most stunning colours can be found outdoors at this time.

Despite the natural beauty, despite your looking forward to the coziness of winter, you find that a few short months later yes, again, things have gone awry. You have ploughed headlong into winter without design or plan; you are wearing the same clothes as last year because you have not put thought into your wardrobe; you have put on weight from indiscriminate eating and you are complaining in your head, or worse, out loud that *'it's cold today'*. This was me!

Many warm-blooded creatures hibernate when it is cold out and go with their natural instincts by doing so. They do not enter the spring season stressed out; rather, animals waking up from hibernation are coming to sleepily, well rested and ready for the warmer season; so, why don't we?

We would not go to sleep for months on end, but perhaps we can take a leaf out of their book and make each winter a mental spa time of rejuvenation, beauty and pleasure.

I decided to write this book as a kind of insurance, to remind me of my exciting winter plans. It is easy to be enthusiastic about the winter season when the leaves are turning. Fall fashions are always fun to look forward to, even for a non-fashionista like me – the September issue of *Vogue*! I can rekindle my love for the colours of plum, navy and camel at this time of year. But a few months later the novelty has already worn off.

This book is also a toolkit of all the ideas that have worked so well in previous winters, as well as new ideas I want to capture. I started this book in autumn, and am now finishing it up in spring. I am so pleased to have tried all my ideas out in a 'test' environment!

This past winter I was working in our retail business. It was raining outside and a customer came in to browse during her lunch break. '*I hate this weather. I hate this time of year*' she complained to me. I commiserated, but after she had gone I felt sad and thought *what a waste of a season.*

We are going to get winter every year whether we like it or not – it's at least a quarter of our life. And that is a good thing. I always think it is better to see another winter than not, don't you?

Please do not wish away the cold season, because that means you are wishing your life away; why not enjoy yourself instead? If you are miserable in the winter, you are setting yourself up to be miserable every year, like clockwork.

Read on to discover my strategy for not just surviving, but *thriving* this winter; on how to have a chic and beautiful winter season and emerge, like a butterfly ready for a gorgeous spring and summer.

Chapter 1.

Know that winter is a different season

Before I wrote this book and became more intentional about the winter months, I sailed into winter every year expecting it to be no different to summer. I assumed things would be the same as the warmer months, but that's how I ended up coming perilously close to being shipwrecked on the rocks of that long, cold, dark time of the year.

Summer is smooth going by comparison, but winter requires special navigational skills. Our bodies react differently and so does our mind.

I have heard that the human body is designed to hold onto weight for insulation during colder weather, which makes sense. In addition, many of us suffer from Seasonal Affective Disorder (S.A.D.) to varying degrees. Are these two factors the reason why we crave sweet treats and simple carbohydrates more than in the summer?

In summer, it is far easier to be healthy. The warm weather and sunshine makes us feel good; we enjoy lighter foods naturally and crave cool water to drink. It is not a hardship to go for a walk after dinner on a beautiful evening, and everything just seems easier when temperatures are mild and the sky is blue.

By contrast, we must look after ourselves in winter, even if we do have a warm, dry home, good healthy food and cozy clothing. I have read studies which show our body's immune system dips, and inflammation rises naturally in the winter, putting us more at risk of inflammatory diseases such as heart disease, rheumatoid arthritis and autoimmune diseases, psychiatric disorders and diabetes.

I was diagnosed as celiac which is also an autoimmune disorder, so this study says I must be even more careful about gluten-containing foods in the winter. I am extremely vigilant anyway, but it is a good reminder to be extra gentle with myself in the cold season.

Winter is the time when we crave comfort foods which can often lead to weight gain. Combine this with the holiday season falling during the northern hemisphere winter and you have the perfect storm for increasing weight if you are not careful.

Because the southern hemisphere winter is mid-year, I purposely have not included anything to do with Christmas in this book. I do, however have a book called '*A Chic and Simple Christmas: Celebrate the holiday season with ease and grace*', which you can find on Amazon here:

https://www.amazon.com/dp/B018UOU68S

Even in the southern hemisphere winter here in New Zealand we are not immune to winter weight gain. Just because our winter covers the middle months of the year does not mean we have it easier.

We might not have Christmas falling in the middle of winter (although the mid-winter Christmas is rather popular as a dinner party theme) but it is still a time when many of us struggle with unhealthy eating, low motivation, sickness, ill health and feeling 'flat'.

Start winter with a goal

When I first had the thought to write this book it was early winter, and I had already gained five kilograms (eleven pounds) since the previous summer season and a few months after this I topped out at ten kilograms (22 pounds) more than my summer low. I did not feel good about this.

I knew it happened every winter and I did overcome it – eventually – *most* years. But my goal is to be a healthy and stable weight year-round, not yo-yo up and down as I had been doing. Yo-yoing doesn't seem to be a particularly *normal* way to be (even though many of us do it), and that is my greatest wish around eating and food – to eat in a *normal* way.

My goal in writing this book was to have a plan to thoroughly enjoy the chilly season and arrive at spring slim and happy, having completed a few interesting and absorbing projects rather than my old not-so-successful coping techniques of blobbing, eating for comfort, and complaining about the cold and/or how inconvenient the weather is.

I wanted to feel trim and healthy under my winter clothes, instead of that nagging feeling that everything was getting tighter (yet I could not find the motivation to change things). For me, the main things I wished to avoid were:

Weight gain

Feeling sluggish

Craving and eating sugary and stodgy foods

No movement – stay on the sofa or at the computer

Feeling a bit flat

Spending most of my time indoors – not much natural light

Throughout this book I am going to address these issues in the way I find most helpful, and that is: instead of focusing on the problem, focus on the opposite – the desired outcome – and then work towards that.

Another way to look at it is to picture an ideal outcome six months down the track and then work backwards on how to make it happen.

An ideal outcome in spring might be:

Being at my ideal weight effortlessly

Feeling like I have enjoyed the winter season

Having had no or very little sickness or ill health

Feeling inspired for the new spring season

Having enjoyed my winter capsule wardrobe and getting dressed each day – I have been creative with my outfits

Perhaps your stress points/goals for winter are like these?

Remember, with anything you need to know, you already have *all the answers* inside of you. Take inspiration from this book or anywhere else and use it as a springboard, but at the same time feel confident that you already know what is best for you.

Be ahead of the game

Instead of waiting until you are deep into the

winter season, have a certain date where you look at your winter planning. Know it is going to be cold and dark and prepare for that.

It may sound obvious, but I would note the leaves turning and admire the beautiful colours of nature, yet block out that part of my mind that would say to me it is obvious winter is on its way. I would still be making my salads for lunch and then be tempted by unhealthy bought lunch options because I had not planned for cold-weather lunches, for example.

Of course, if it is already mid-winter, know that you can turn things around and that it is not too late. If this is the case, the best time to start is *today*, not tomorrow, and not next winter. You can turn things around in an instant when you decide to.

Areas to plan for are:

Healthy winter meals that are simple and delicious

Making your home cozy and appealing for winter

Creating your winter capsule wardrobe

Having a project or two that you would like to complete

Feeling like you have been active in an enjoyable way

Keeping healthy and buoyant of mind

I have put all my research and everything I have learned into this one book – which will be extremely helpful next winter, when I will likely have forgotten what worked well!

I hope it proves useful to you also and that you find appealing and inspirational ideas in these pages.

Look forward to winter

When you think about it logically, there is no point in complaining about winter or hating the fact that it is cold every year. You can't change that. Instead, look at all the positives of the season. Plan for and enjoy the enforced downtime when the weather is rough. Don't wish your life away by being miserable at least three months of every year.

Be excited for a season to cocoon. This is not hard for me as I love being cozy inside.

Think of all the good things you can do during winter, *without guilt* since you cannot go outside as much.

Do you have childhood memories of being told to go outside and play in the sunshine and that it is a waste to be indoors? I do! That's why it feels like such a treat to me to cozy up inside in the winter.

I love at-home activities such as reading, craft-work, journaling, baking, putting on casseroles or the slow-cooker, and making soup. Equally though, I love rugging up and going for a crisp, clear walk in the winter sunshine, or with an umbrella if there is spitty rain.

Wintry highlights for me include:

Lighting candles every day. They do not have to be expensive – tealights look so pretty in a glass jar. If I am at home writing for the day I like to choose one of my scented candles and light it on my desk. I am paranoid about one of our two cats knocking it if I leave the room, so if I go to do a job such as hanging out the washing or going for a walk, I blow the candle out.

Having a candle flame in view is a simple and easy way to feel cozy. It feels like a treat and as if someone is taking care of you. I know that sounds strange but I'm sure you know what I mean. Because a candle is not a necessity (unless you have a power cut), they feel nurturing, special and a little bit luxurious.

Books and magazines. I love having a selection of books and magazines to look forward to – I visit the library each week and I also have a never-ending supply of my own at home (I truly don't know how I come by them all, they just seem to turn up, book-magpie that I am).

With magazines, I love to change my reading material out. I have a few titles that I keep because I know I will re-read them over and over (such as *Victoria*) and they don't take up much room. I like to get out the winter issues and have them displayed so that I have seasonal reading to feel cozy and inspired.

A craft project. Something that makes me excited for the upcoming winter season is to choose a craft project I would like to complete. I usually pick something portable so that I can have guilt-free sofa time with a movie or television programme each night. With this consistent progress, my project is soon finished.

I might choose to knit a scarf, house slippers

or a baby gift. Hand-sewn patchwork items and needlepoint projects are also great. Small projects are my preferred option. This past winter I discovered the lovely cross-stitch patterns at Peacock & Fig (https://peacockandfig.com/) – there are cute free patterns and small projects such as an eyeglass case, pin cushion and coffee sleeve among others.

When a project is too big it can be daunting, and no-one wants to bring out a half-finished project the following winter; both the novelty and your enthusiasm have probably worn off by then. It always feels better to start a project that you know you have a chance of finishing.

Journaling. I love to plan and dream in my journal, and winter is a perfect time to do this. I have a few different journals on the go – one is for goal lists, writing and blog ideas and to note down quotes I love. This one travels everywhere in my handbag so it looks a little battered now that it is almost full.

I also have prettier journals that I keep in my bedside drawers, and these are used to dream, list out details of my perfect life and write my future into reality. I do write in the summer as well, but there is something about a rainy afternoon at home that begs for a little journaling time. I also go to bed earlier in the winter, and usually spend some time on the bed writing in one of my journals before I go to sleep.

Cooking and baking. Often on a cold winter's day I start thinking about dinner at breakfast-time, which is when I get my slow cooker out. I am inspired to chop vegetables aplenty and layer them in with diced meat and flavourings to simmer away all day. The bonus on top of a delicious dinner is that, later in the day when I would normally have to start cooking, dinner has already been made.

What are your favourite winter comforts? Collect them for inspiration during the dark cold days to ensure that you comfort yourself in ways other than just with food.

Chapter 2.

Create a winter menu plan

The first thing I started thinking about for my *Chic Winter* plan was food, because it was my biggest stumbling block.

Don't make the mistake I have made in the past of not acknowledging winter. I was on a good streak of salads for summer lunches and I enjoyed them a lot. As autumn turned into winter though, I was still making salads. I wasn't paying attention to the weather and ended up having salads for lunch and resenting them, or buying unhealthy and expensive hot lunch foods when the day was simply too cold and rainy for a salad.

That was when I realised I had *no winter menu plan.* So, I made a list of our favourite meals that were portable and suitable for a lunch at work, and lunches that were quick and easy to have at home.

I asked myself, '*what are some great lunch ideas that are going to keep me happy and healthily nourished*'. I wanted them to be simple to prepare, easy to heat up and not too expensive either. I started putting together my winter lunch menu for the season – sort of like a capsule clothing collection, but it's your capsule *menu* collection instead.

When I have the idea of cooking an old favourite, I search for recipes online to get a general idea of the recipe. I don't usually follow a recipe to the letter; more often I will merge a few together and tweak them to suit my dietary requirements and what I have in the kitchen, as well as making them as healthy as possible without sacrificing taste too much.

Start a notebook of *your* favourite winter meals. They don't have to be recipes if you already have dishes that you have cooked a million times before; just make a note of the dish. I find I forget seasonal recipes from year to year and slip into easier and less healthy options, so just noting down the meal outline jogs my memory to include that in our repertoire.

Think about your favourite winter meals (dividing into breakfast, lunch and dinner). Browse Pinterest or recipe Web sites online for inspiration. Save your favourites.

By having a menu ready from last winter for example, it's as easy as choosing in a restaurant, because I often find coming up with ideas is the most challenging part of cooking meals.

The main thing for me was to make the healthy stuff desirable so that I wasn't tempted by simple and stodgy carbohydrate cravings. The bad stuff might feel like a treat at the time, but afterwards you feel worse and put on weight; it can be a downward spiral.

There is a great saying that summer bodies are made in winter. Keeping this in mind helps me look for healthy meals in the winter and drink hot peppermint tea instead of snacking on chocolate when I am bored.

Breakfasts that are warming, filling and healthy

Breakfasts are easy for me in the summer. I love fresh, chopped seasonal fruit with a spoonful of Greek yoghurt and a handful of raw mixed nuts on top. With a homemade milky coffee for afters, I am set until lunchtime.

We do still have fruit for breakfast a lot in the winter, but some mornings you need something hot. My less healthy winter breakfasts used to consist of toast with butter and jam or peanut butter, and rolled oats with brown sugar and cream.

I changed to fresh fruit because I wanted to eat healthier, but then I thought, why not make my winter favourites more nutritious so I can still enjoy them *and* be slim?

I tried cooking oats with fresh fruit, and it was delicious. Pear worked the best, so I would simmer oats on the stove with pieces of chopped pair (I washed them and left the skin on), with a handful of raisins and a tiny sprinkle of cinnamon. These ingredients made the oats sweet enough for me so that I didn't want brown sugar, although you could add some honey or sugar if you wanted to.

It might take a few more minutes to prepare than a sachet of flavoured oats, but the taste of real food is far preferable, and you know that real ingredients equal a happy body and a happy mind. I often crave warm and 'stodgy' when it is wintry outside and this breakfast provides both, along with good health.

My way to healthy up my winter toast was to have two-soft boiled eggs on a piece of buttered toast. This breakfast is quick to make – bring the eggs to the boil in a small pot of water, then boil for 3.5 minutes. Cool in cold water for a few minutes and peel while your toast is down. They are like poached eggs, but I find them far easier to cook and you waste less of the precious white as well (which is where all the protein is).

You might feel like I did and think that you would rather have something sweet on your toast, but after you've had your eggs, a sweet taste is the last thing on your mind. Who knew that protein fixes sugar cravings – hoorah!

Both these healthy winter breakfasts keep me full until lunchtime and they are delicious and satisfying to eat. All the ingredients are easy to find, not too expensive and simple to keep at home too.

What are your favourite breakfasts? How could you 'winterize' them and make them healthier at the same time?

Lunches for work and home

As winter advanced, I very quickly realized that I needed to create warming and healthy winter lunches. I love a big salad with protein in the summer, but as I mentioned at the beginning of this chapter, last winter I did not plan, ending up either freezing cold eating cold salad for lunch (très depressing) or buying something stodgy and hot (not slimming).

I wanted to create a bank of healthy, cozy and warming winter lunch ideas and simple recipes that I could take to work to heat up with a side salad. Along the lines of frittata, soup, oven bakes etc.

Winter lunches were the meals that were most challenging for me. Having a choice of healthy salad or unhealthy bought lunch were options that were poles apart. I was too black-and-white in my thinking though, because I would tell myself that I could either have a healthy salad, or my only alternative was to buy something unhealthy, high-carb and fatty. It seems silly when I say it out loud, but in my mind at the time, a salad was the only healthy option.

Because my husband and I work together in our retail business, we mostly eat the same lunches. We had a brainstorming session coming up with good ideas for winter lunches we could bring from home and heat up. We remembered successful lunch ideas from previous winters and noted those down too.

On our list were items such as:

Frittata
Soup
Bolognese/Savoury mince
Individual cottage pies
Chicken curry
Casserole hotpot
Mini pizzas made with corn-wraps as a base

I still love to have a side salad with my hot lunch, but my husband is not a fan in winter. He will either have his lunch as is, or sometimes adds a cup of frozen vegetables to bulk up his portion. To make sure I get my salads in, I will make a couple of days' worth at a time, then all I have to do is open the container and tip it into a bowl. Being washed and chopped ahead of time makes the side salad extra crispy and delicious too.

Most workplaces have a microwave. You could invest in a few glass or microwave-safe plastic dishes with snap-on lids, and take a portion to work each day. Even taking the bus I used to carry lunch items to work sometimes. You might add vegetables to your hot dish, or you may be like me and prefer a crunchy side salad to go with it, which is easy to prepare the night before and put in a small Tupperware container in the fridge.

Make up a big batch of whatever you choose on the Sunday and you are set for a week of yummy, healthy and inexpensive lunches. You might decide to have homemade lunches Monday to Thursday and buy yourself lunch as a treat on a Friday.

You can have dinner leftovers and store a couple of extras each week in the freezer too; that way you have an instant lunch – just take the container out of the freezer and put it in the fridge the night before. If you make 1-2 extra each week you can have a week off lunch prep every so often, or ready options when you get busy and have no lunch prepared. Back-up lunches in the freezer are a great find at times like this.

Because we also store homemade dinners in the freezer, I keep a roll of masking tape and a permanent marker in the kitchen. It's quick and easy to tear off a piece of tape and stick on the lid, then write the meal name down. I started doing this when I realised *everything* looks the same when it is frozen. Masking tape is easy to peel off when you go to wash the container as well.

Dinners – tweak the winter classics

Winter is the easiest time to cook at home. It is just less appealing to go out to eat when it is cold and rainy. Winter evenings *beg* for an oven-cooked meal and there are so many warm and comforting dinners that can be made healthier – soups, casseroles, slow-cooked meals, roasts and shepherd's pie are some of my favourites.

The trick is to choose meals that are comforting and healthy and contain enough protein without being too high in fat or carbs. The alternative is to make your favourite meals healthier – roasts with lots of vegetables (not as many starchy), not adding fat or oil to the pan, tipping off the roasting fat to make gravy, etc.

Our winter menu often includes these dishes:

Roast chicken, beef or lamb
Crumbed chicken pieces or chicken breast as a mini-roast
Shepherd's pie
Spaghetti Bolognese
Pasta or rice bake
'Bangers' (sausages) and mash
Parmesan chicken

Our oven gets a lot of use in the winter – 6-7 times per week we use it in preference to stove-top. It's just so easy to assemble everything, put it in the oven, set the timer and forget about it until the buzzer goes off.

In the winter, I love to spend a bit of time in the kitchen making bigger quantities of food than normal, then at mealtimes I have a ready-made meal. There are boutique cafes and food stores that offer fresh, chilled gourmet ready-meals and the prices can be quite high for a single or double serving. So why not make your own?

With a few Gladware or Tupperware containers you can easily replicate these gourmet ready-meals at a much lower cost *and* with ingredients to suit your taste and any preferences or health issues.

Recently I chopped and prepped vegetables for an hour, and the beautiful result is a huge pot of soup which will be lunch for the next week, and a pasta bake which will do at least two or three evening meals for us both (and my husband is a big eater).

I love to have an interesting audio going on my phone or iPod and the chopping time passes by in a pleasant way. Alternatively, I might have music playing – opera is great to get into the mood to make Italian food.

We don't tend to have desserts on an ordinary evening, instead finishing off our meal with a coffee or tea and bliss ball or a piece or two of dark chocolate. When we do have guests however, I think I make a crumble every time. What can I say, it's my favourite dessert – and my husband's too.

Snacks

In an ideal world, I prefer not to snack so much, instead getting the bulk of my nourishment from my three main meals. I always keep healthy snack options available though; that way there is always something if I am hungry. Late afternoon is the only 'official' snack time for me, and I don't eat something every day at this time, only if I find myself hungry.

My snack options include:

Fresh fruit that is portable such as bananas or mandarins
Raw nuts
A bliss ball
A small quantity of cheese and rice crackers

For example, I might take a banana to work and have this with several raw almonds later in the afternoon if I know dinner is still a few hours away. Or if I am at home, it is a treat to sit down with a book or magazine and half-a-dozen rice crackers with thin slivers of brie on top.

I discovered bliss balls this year and love them. They are a sweet treat which are also packed with protein and nutrients. They are made with real ingredients and keep for a while too. My own version is in the recipe section at the end of this chapter, and I also buy *Frooz Balls* (despite the terrible name) which are a New Zealand-made bliss ball when I haven't been organized enough to make any.

Drinks count as snacks for me too, even though they aren't food. Often it is a rest that I want, so I will make a hot drink and enjoy that whilst taking a break. I love Earl Grey or English Breakfast tea with trim milk, or coffee with creamy milk (no sugar in either, thank you).

Alternatively, I might pour a champagne flute of Perrier sparkling mineral water in Lemon or Lime flavour later in the day. These are delicious and don't seem to have any calories, yet are just as nice to me (if not nicer) than flavoured drinks.

Fiona's favourite winter recipes

I am so happy to share with you my staples of everyday health and happiness in the winter. Take them, try them, adapt them to your own tastes and start your own winter capsule menu plan for this year; then revisit next year and tweak as you go to ensure they become firm family favourites.

Red Lentil and Tomato soup

Don't be put off by the word 'lentil' in this recipe. I usually bypass any recipe with the that word (unfair as it sounds) but this is not your usual lentil recipe. Think 'rustic Italian meal in a bowl' instead of 'brown health food from the 1970s'.

You will need:

1 onion, chopped and sautéed in one tablespoon of olive oil

1 400g (14 oz.) can of plain or flavoured chopped tomatoes and juice

1 cup red lentils (rinsed and picked over – take out the odd yucky looking one)

4 cups/1 litre/1-quart chicken stock (or any other stock flavour you like). I use a mix of

homemade chicken stock and store-bought stock powder/cubes.

(In my head, the recipe is: one onion, 1 can tomatoes, 1 cup red lentils, 1 litre stock – easy to remember). All the basic recipe ingredients are 'store cupboard ingredients' which means they are easy to keep on hand.

After sautéing the onion, add everything to the pot, bring to the boil and simmer for twenty minutes. That's it!

This soup has been one of my staple lunches both at work and home for many winters. It reheats beautifully in the microwave and I have even been known to make it before work (when I have no extra time). The quick version involves throwing the onion into the other ingredients without sautéing and then cooking for 20 minutes. If you are pressed for time you could use the stock, a can of flavoured tomatoes and the red lentils, no onion.

You can also add extras to this recipe if you desire, to create different flavours. Additions that I have tried which taste delicious are:

Tiny dice of celery and carrot, sautéed with the onion to add flavour. This trio is known as *mirepoix*. According to Google, '*mirepoix* is the

French culinary term for a combination of diced carrots, onions and celery sautéed in butter and used as an aromatic base to flavour sauces, soups and stews. Even a small amount can significantly contribute to the overall flavour of a finished dish'. Since I learned about *mirepoix* I have been using it a lot. I feel very European doing so!

A handful of fresh pumpkin cubes. These cook within the twenty-minute time frame and you can break up the pieces with a potato masher when done. It is a nicer soup a little rustic than pureed smooth, I feel.

Any fresh vegetables that are languishing tired in your fridge can be chopped up small (since you're not pureeing) and added to the mix as it cooks.

Fresh or dried herbs to tweak the flavour in any direction. I have successfully used fresh oregano from my garden (tear the leaves off the stem once washed), dried sweet basil and bay leaves (remove bay leaves after cooking).

A little tomato paste to intensify the flavour. You might have a small amount left over in the fridge that you want to use up, or a few cubes in the freezer you'd like to clear out.

Any cooked meats if you like, however the lentils provide good protein so it is not strictly needed for a balanced meal. But imagine a small piece of leftover steak diced up and added to the soup near the end, or leftover shredded roast chicken. Delicious!

Full-fat plain, unsweetened or Greek yoghurt – just a dollop – added before serving is divine.

A sprinkle of Parmesan if you are going for an Italian vibe is delicious too.

Flavoured tomatoes or spices for a different flavour type – i.e. Italian, Mexican or Indian.

Another particularly delicious batch of this soup included pumpkin as above, combined with Indian-flavoured chopped tomatoes and an extra teaspoon of yellow curry powder.

I rarely make a single batch of this soup. Doubling the quantities does not take much more effort, and I often freeze the second container for an instant week's worth of lunches.

Pumpkin Soup

1 onion

2 garlic cloves

1 tablespoon of olive oil or butter

Pumpkin – half of a small pumpkin or one quarter if your pumpkin is huge

In a soup pot or your largest pot, sauté onion and garlic in olive oil/butter (or both, it is delicious using a little of each). Add one-inch cubes of any kind of peeled and seeded pumpkin and then top up to the level of pumpkin with homemade or bought chicken or vegetable stock.

Simmer for twenty minutes or until pumpkin is soft. Leave your soup in the pot but turn off the heat. Either use a potato masher in the pot for a chunky soup or a stick/immersion blender for a smooth soup. You can also use a blender to puree. I prefer my pumpkin soup to be smooth.

This is where you can add seasonings, trim milk, cream or even coconut milk. You can add any types of flavourings to give your soup a different flavour each time i.e. thyme with cream, Thai herbs and chilli flakes with coconut milk, or a teaspoon of yellow curry powder.

A fine dining restaurant I worked at as a teen served their pumpkin soup with a teaspoon of roasted, salted cashew nuts on top. I still remember how delicious that combination was.

Vegetable soup

1 kumara (sweet potato)

¼ pumpkin

½ onion

1 clove of garlic

1 carrot

1 courgette (zucchini)

1 leek

1 stalk of celery

Peel, wash and chop vegetables where applicable. Slice or dice onions finely and chop vegetables into one-inch cubes. Fill a soup or stock pot to half way with vegetables and fill the pot to three quarters with hot water. Add the appropriate amount of stock seasoning (I use four *Massel* stock cubes for the size of my pot) and anything else you'd like. For example, sometimes I add a heaped teaspoon of yellow curry powder for a mellow warming taste and other times it might be mixed dried herbs.

Once everything is soft, use an immersion blender to puree. Top up with hot water to adjust the thickness to your preference. If you want to sauté the onions and celery first in olive oil and/or butter you can, but I haven't been doing this lately and the soup is just as delicious.

Serve with a decent-sized dollop of Greek yoghurt or sour cream and a sprinkling of fresh cut parsley (optional).

Spaghetti Bolognese
Savoury mince
Shepherd's pie

To keep my life simple, I have one base recipe for beef mince that I know off by heart, which, when tweaked in the right direction, becomes any of the above. I know purists would not be happy with this method but that's okay, I am not going for a cooking award.

To begin with, sauté:

1 onion

1 celery stalk

1 carrot

(all three finely diced)

1 tablespoon of olive oil

1 stock cube

Cook these ingredients on a low heat in a frying pan or *Le Crueset*-type metal dish. As the stock cube softens, spread it into the vegetables, stirring around with a wooden spoon, and let everything caramelize together. Add 500g (1 pound) of lean beef mince and brown with the vegetables. Then add a can of tomatoes (400g/14 oz.) and either a sachet of gravy mix (use 'simmer' rather than 'instant') or a couple of teaspoons of cornflour mixed with a small amount of cold water.

Add 6 finely sliced mushrooms and stir the whole mix thoroughly, then let it simmer on a low heat for about twenty minutes.

To make spaghetti Bolognese:
Add Italian dried herbs, or fresh parsley and oregano; serve over pasta with a sprinkling of Parmesan cheese.

To make savoury mince:
Add a few drops of Worcestershire sauce and serve with noodles or mashed potato and vegetables.

To make shepherd's pie:
Place in a ceramic dish with high sides, top with mashed potato and heat in the oven until the potato is slightly browned on top and the sauce is bubbling up around the edges. Serve with baby peas and gravy.

There are even more options with this base recipe:

Pot pie:
Spoon into individual pie dishes or ramekins, top with a round of ready-made rolled flaky pastry and heat in the oven until the pastry is golden. Serve with hot chips (French fries) or a baked potato and vegetables or salad.

Any of the above are great for lunch servings too. If I am in a hurry in the morning, I take a small portion of the basic recipe to heat up for my lunch at work, and grab a carrot out of the vegetable drawer. It is not exactly an elegant lunch, but it is tasty, healthy, warming, high in protein and most importantly at this time, quick.

Roast chicken

We have roast chicken at least once a week. It is so easy to make and a delicious meal. You will need:

1 fresh chicken

Roasting vegetables – we usually use 3 or 4 of onion, carrot, potato, pumpkin and kumara (sweet potato).

Steaming vegetables – maybe broccoli, cauliflower, green beans or frozen baby peas. We will usually have two of these.

Place the chicken on its back in a large roasting dish and put into a moderate oven (180 deg C, 350 deg F). There is no need to add any extra oil, fat or butter. After half an hour, take the roasting pan out of the oven and tilt so that the fat released spreads over the base of the pan. Place vegetables around the chicken. In total, the chicken usually takes 1.5 hours and the vegetables take one hour, turning half-way through. The exact cooking time will vary per the size of your chicken, so check the packaging for the time you need.

When everything is ready, turn off the oven. Place the chicken on a plate or chopping board and cover with foil and a tea towel to keep warm. Transfer all the roast vegetables to another oven dish and put them back in the oven to keep warm.

Tip all the fat from the roasting pan into a tin. I always save an empty tin and keep it in the fridge, filling up with fat from each roast and throwing in the rubbish once it is full. Do not tip fat down the sink or your drain may block once the fat solidifies – ask me how I know that!

Place the roasting pan on a stove-top element on low-moderate heat.

To make the gravy I use *Orgran* gravy powder, mixing two tablespoons into a cup of cold water with a fork. Tip liquid into the roasting dish and stir gently with a wooden spatula, scraping up all the lovely caramelized bits of chicken and vegetables.

Once the gravy has thickened, tip it into a jug and serve over your roast meal. While I am doing the gravy, my husband carves the chicken and I serve up the vegetables.

If you don't want to roast a whole chicken, you can do a mini-roast by using chicken breasts or bone-in chicken pieces. Allow an hour in total, so meat and vegetables can go in at the same. If you are using chicken breasts, make a little lid of tin foil and place over the chicken breasts and tuck it around them to stop them drying out. Turn the chicken breasts/pieces when you turn the vegetables and they will get lovely and brown on both sides.

'Bangers' (sausages) and mash

This is a yummy treat meal that has virtually no preparation time. We don't have it a lot because sausages aren't as good for you as other meat options, even when you choose the healthy, gourmet ones. There are still nitrates in them that you don't want to have too often. But, being from English heritage, I do love a bangers and mash meal once a month or so.

Choose nice-quality sausages and put them in a cold frying pan, no added fat or oil. I usually have one for myself, and my husband has two. Turn the element on low and let them heat slowly. I read this advice on a gourmet sausage packet – 'cook these low and slow' and I always remember that now when I cook sausages. When you cook them this way they release their own fat to cook in. Once they are browned on one side, turn them over and add a finely diced onion to the pan, stirring around to soak in all that yummy sausage goodness.

I leave the sausages and onion on low the whole cooking time and place a lid on the pan, so the moisture stays in and the onions caramelize rather than catch and burn. Turn the sausages occasionally so they brown on all sides and stir the onion around at the same time.

In the meantime, boil Agria or similar floury/golden (not waxy) potatoes (1-2 per person, depending on their size) in salty water, then mash with a tablespoon of milk and a tablespoon of butter. Optional: fresh chopped parsley is delicious in mashed potatoes. Keep warm in the pot until the sausages are ready.

Steam or boil baby peas to go with this meal and lastly, once the sausage and onion mix is cooked, tip a simmer gravy into the pan and stir through to coat everything and pick up the delicious caught bits on the bottom of the pan. I do this while the sausages and onion are still in the pan, using two tablespoons of *Orgran* gravy mix with either one cup of water or one cup of *Campbell's* liquid beef stock. You can use any packet of 'simmer' gravy. This will thicken up within a few minutes.

Serve the sausages on top of the mash, peas

on the side and pour your onion gravy over the top. Serve up to a very happy family!

Parmesan chicken

1 chicken breast per person (I have a half-breast if they are large)

¼ cup of breadcrumbs

1 clove garlic

2 tablespoons of shredded Parmesan cheese

Seasoning such as chicken salt or garlic salt

Optional: fresh herbs if you have them around, such as parsley, thyme or oregano (washed and dried)

I have a Cuisinart 'Mini Prep' tiny food processor which is great for making crumb mixes, but you can just as easily mix them together without one.

Combine everything in the food processor and pulse until combined and the garlic is minced. Tip into a clean plastic bag with your chicken breasts and shake until the chicken is coated.

If you don't have a food processor, tip the

breadcrumbs into a plastic bag and begin adding everything else – chop the garlic finely, add Parmesan, sprinkle in seasoning and tip in chopped herbs, then shake as above.

Line an oven tray with baking paper and spray lightly with olive oil. Place chicken breasts on paper and bake in the oven at 180 deg C or 350 deg F for about fifty minutes, turning thirty minutes in.

We often have this meal with no starchy vegetables, although you could easily cook potatoes in the oven at the same time. A nice Italian-style side would be diced potato cooked in a dish sprayed or tossed with olive oil and Italian herbs and chicken salt seasoning. We have fresh rosemary in our garden which I finely chop and sprinkle over roasting potato and it smells and tastes amazing.

In the last ten minutes of cooking time, steam your vegetables – any combination of cauliflower, broccoli, green beans, carrots, asparagus or peas depending what is in season.

Once the vegetables are turned on to steam, prepare your sauce – add two tablespoons of cornflour to a 400g (14 oz.) can of diced tomatoes (plain or Italian-flavoured), season to taste, and simmer for five minutes or until bubbling and thickened. Stir with a whisk as it heats. Serve over chicken breast and vegetables. Fresh chopped parsley is delicious in this sauce and adds a wonderful contrast of colour.

Crumbed chicken

Our weekday mini-roast is one of our staple meals.

Skinless chicken thigh cutlets (one for me, two for my husband)

1 heaped teaspoon of Sweet Spanish paprika

¼ cup of breadcrumbs

A sprinkle of chicken salt (or normal salt)

½ teaspoon of mustard powder or ginger

Combine everything in a plastic bag and shake until the chicken pieces are coated. I use baking paper to cook this meal and it helps with pan clean-up. You don't get much for gravy from crumbed chicken, so I tend to serve with gravy mix rather than pan gravy.

Bake everything in a moderate 180 deg C, 350 deg F oven for fifty minutes, turning after thirty minutes. Steam vegetables in the last ten minutes and use the boiling water to make instant gravy.

Pasta Bake

Sunday evenings to me spell something comforting in the kitchen. Often this means an Italian dish such as pasta bake.

This dish can be made lighter than a traditional pasta bake by adding more vegetables and less pasta. I also use cottage cheese instead of béchamel or ricotta. Cottage cheese still tastes delicious but is low in fat and high in protein.

I love this meal because it is comfort food, and it is also a dish I can compile everything at once, put it in the oven for an hour or two and sit down with a book. The aroma as it cooks is mouth-watering.

Here is my recipe:

In a deep lasagne or casserole dish add the following in layers (you don't need to worry about greasing or oiling the dish, just pile everything in).

Mix together the bottom layer in a big bowl:

Diced pumpkin (1-inch cubes)

Silver beet (chard), washed and chopped

One onion, chopped

1-2 cloves garlic, crushed and chopped

500g (about 1 lb.) cottage cheese

Seasoning - plenty of salt and pepper, sweet smoked paprika, chicken stock powder, dried chilli flakes and rubbed sage. Use any combo that you have in your pantry.

With the first layer, you can combine any vegetables you want to use up; I always include pumpkin as it imparts a rich sweetness and thickens the pasta bake. You can use a small container of cottage cheese if you have a smaller dish.

Second layer, sprinkle mozzarella cheese and then add dried, uncooked pasta. I see no point in having to cook pasta first. You can use lasagne sheets, but all I had was macaroni elbows for my most recent pasta bake and they worked just fine. Use enough to cover the cheese in a single layer.

Third layer, pour a can or two of diced tomatoes over, spreading out the tomato pieces. Rinse out the can(s) with the tiniest amount of water and pour this in too. This time I added a splash of red wine (just into the middle of the mix, and let it soak in) as I thought there might not have been quite enough liquid. You don't want too much liquid though, just enough to absorb into the pasta.

Fourth and final layer, add another generous sprinkle of mozzarella cheese. A sprinkle of Parmesan is nice too. Finally, top with breadcrumbs. You can use store-bought or homemade. Optional: tip the breadcrumbs into a food processor, add a clove or two of garlic and any seasoning you like and blitz.

Sprinkle breadcrumbs on the top (hopefully you haven't reached the rim of the dish) and place in a moderate 180 deg C, 350 deg F oven for at least 1.5 hours. Cover the dish with tin foil for the first half, then take off for the second half.

When you want to check that your pasta bake is ready, stick a fork in it and check that the pumpkin is soft, and try a piece of the pasta to ensure it is cooked. There should be a nice, thick consistency too – if you see runny liquid on the top, cook a little longer until it is all evaporated.

You can add a side salad to this if you like, but we often go for the 'scurvy' option and rely on the vegetables in the dish itself for our nutrients.

Pasta bake makes great leftovers for lunch at work. Once it cools overnight in the fridge, it is easy to slice into pieces which can then be heated up in the microwave.

Rice Bake

One night I went to make a pasta bake and realised that I didn't have a single piece, not even one, of pasta in the house when I went to use it. I wasn't about to go out just for that (even though it's quite a main ingredient in pasta bake...), so I substituted rice. My reasoning was that risotto is Italian and it has rice in it rather than pasta.

My husband was dubious at best but raved about it afterwards. Here is the recipe for my accidental rice bake:

500g (1 pound) lean beef mince

1 400g (14 oz.) can chopped tomatoes and juice. Rinse the can out with a small amount of water - less than 1/4 can) and mix this in too.

Seasoning. Sometimes I get fancy and make it up myself and sometimes I use packets. Lately I have been using:

1 pkt *Simply Organic* Mushroom Sauce mix

1 pkt *Simply Organic* Tomato Basil Spaghetti Sauce mix

1 large 500g (18 oz.) tub of cottage cheese

1 cup of rice, rinsed in a sieve

½ onion chopped

Small amounts of kumara and pumpkin in tiny dice

10 mushrooms chopped

Mix everything together and spoon into a rectangular oven dish which has been wiped over with olive oil and a paper towel (or cooking spray).

Cover with foil and bake at 180 deg C, 350 deg F for an hour. Take the foil off, grate some cheese over the top and return to the oven for half an hour. I love meals like this where all the preparation is at the beginning and you can relax while it cooks.

When your rice bake is ready it should be lightly browned on the top with all liquid absorbed. Check near the end to make sure it is not getting too dark and dry. Or, if it is still quite liquidy, cook for a little while longer – check every 10-15 minutes.

As with the pasta bake, this dish reheats well

for lunches.

Apple and Boysenberry Crumble

3 granny smith apples, peeled, cored and sliced – place in a ceramic oven dish

1 425g/15oz. can of boysenberries in syrup, poured over the apple slices and mixed around – use the syrup too

You could use different fruits or just go with the classic Apple Crumble by using 4-6 granny smith apples by themselves. If using fresh apples only, I would dot with 6-8 small cubes of butter and sprinkle with a little bit of brown sugar. You will only want to use granny smith apples (they are green and quite tart) because they are far nicer than using sweet red apples in hot desserts.

Crumble topping:

1/2 cup flour (I used a gluten-free flour mix but you could use normal plain flour)

1/2 cup almond meal

2 tablespoons coconut flakes or desiccated

coconut (optional)

2-4 tablespoons cubed cold butter, dice-size

2 tablespoons brown sugar

1 teaspoon cinnamon

Pulse the crumble mixture briefly in a food processor until it resembles the texture of uneven and lumpy rubble. You do not want to blend it until it is completely smooth. Alternatively rub the butter into the flour and then mix in the other ingredients.

Spread the crumble topping over the fruit and bake in a moderate oven (180C/350F) for 30-40 minutes. When the crumble is ready it will be golden brown and have fruit juice bubbling around the edges of the dish. Serve with vanilla ice-cream, custard or whipped cream.

Bliss Balls

1 cup dates

1/2 cup dried apricots

1 cup almond meal

2 tablespoons coconut flakes (or desiccated)

1 tablespoon coconut oil (optional)

1-2 tablespoons peanut butter

Whizz the dates and apricots in a food processor, then add the other ingredients and whizz again. Roll into balls and coat in desiccated coconut. I store mine in the fridge which makes them nice and chewy, but they don't have to be refrigerated.

This quantity of ingredients makes about thirteen decent-sized bliss balls.

I used coconut oil because I already had a jar, however I've only ever put it on my face before, not in my food. I know coconut oil has excellent health-giving qualities, so I'm happy to have found a way to eat it.

These are a great alternative to dark chocolate for after meals. Yes, bliss balls are high in fat and sugar, but you only eat one as a serving. They wouldn't be so healthy if you ate quite a few at once, but then you probably wouldn't want to because they are rich and satisfying. Even though they are healthy, they are still a treat food.

Chapter 3.

Break up the long winter

I think the thing with winter is that we go into it with the expectation of a long, cold, dark season more or less, depending on where we live. Some places have a dry season and a rainy season instead of a warm season and a cool season, but the thought is the same – winter is generally a time to 'get through' so that we can enjoy our summer on the other side.

Instead of blobbing on the couch, which let's face it, is very easy to get into the habit of; why not plan a few outings, occasions or even a vacation to punctuate the winter season.

Being a home-loving introvert, hibernating at home with the fire going and a good television programme, movie or book is my favourite way to spend a winter evening; however even I can get cabin fever and feel like winter is closing in on me, never to end.

Going to see a movie at the theatre is fun, and it breaks up a routine week. Buy your tickets ahead of time so you are not tempted to flake out on your plans. The last time we saw a movie we bought the tickets when we were passing the theatre during the day. Later on that evening, we both grumbled and moaned and said to each other 'wish we hadn't bought those tickets'. We went though (of course); the movie was wonderful; the renovated boutique theatre was a lovely place to be; the other patrons were elegantly refined, and our evening turned out fun and energising.

If you have the time and money available, why not **plan for a mid-winter break?** I long to do this one day, because I have never had a beach holiday in the middle of winter before. Here in New Zealand it is popular to go to Fiji, Tahiti and other Pacific islands. Australian destinations such as the Gold Coast and Noosa are very popular too and a bit further afield for us is Bali or Thailand.

I vow to myself that within the next couple of years, we will save up for a mid-winter holiday and in the meantime, I can look forward to it and research places to go. Whenever someone mentions that they have just been on a holiday, I quiz them on where they went. Where exactly was it? Would they recommend the area, the resort? I make notes and not only does it get me excited for our beach holiday to come, but I gather valuable information.

If a mid-winter vacation is not on the cards for you, can you have a weekend or even a week-long staycation? Plan for it and book it in just like a normal vacation, except that your travel time and cost is zero, and accommodation costs you no extra either. If you can book annual leave from your job, so much the better.

Have your home clean and tidy before your staycation, then enjoy a fun, chore-free time. You could:

- Be a tourist in your own town.

- Go out for lunch.

- Have yummy foods – plan for easy and simple meals, eat out or have takeaway food for a treat.

- Go to a movie or have a movie day at home.

- Go on a zoo outing.

- Go for a day walk if the weather is fine.

- Visit an area for a walk around and a coffee, such as the waterfront or a similar touristy area where you live. As a local you probably never do these things, but when you do, it feels like you are on holiday when you mingle with the tourists.

- Go for a hot swim and spa at your local pool.

If spending time off work doing nothing but enjoying yourself sounds far too decadent, how about planning a job that keeps getting put off; for example, cleaning out the garage or painting your living room. Budget one or two days for that and have a strict finishing time; then enjoy the next few days' staycation as a reward and a 'well done' for your hard work.

You will have something to celebrate; you will be looking forward to relaxing; you will feel satisfied having completed a big job *and* you will have the bonus of a 'new' garage, living room or whatever project you have done. I counted all the benefits, and you have a win/win/win/win right there.

Learn something or have a project to complete

What could you learn or achieve that is fun this winter? Think about something you have always wanted to do, but never gotten around to. Why not set yourself an enticing 'winter school' project and dive right in? Perhaps you would like to:

- Go to a night class
- Sew something simple, such as a skirt for summer
- Learn a language
- Read a classic book
- Study art history
- Practice needlepoint or cross-stitch
- Do a personal development course
- Make an infinity scarf if you are a knitter
- Small indoor home improvements
- Write a book

- Declutter your closet or junk room

Write a list of projects you would love to complete during the winter months. Pick one thing from the list that excites you and it will not be a chore to set aside a couple of hours each week to learn or work towards.

Refer to this list when you are feeling blah and unmotivated and choose the item that looks the most fun and easy to focus on. Getting your creativity going helps you forget about the fact that winter can be a depressing time, and you will feel much satisfaction coming into spring with at least one completed project. Look forward to that good feeling when you are getting started.

I know I have things like this on my wish-list that I haven't done, simply because I haven't done them. I just let them float along on that list for years. Some of them I know deep down I don't care whether I do them or not, but some are real interests that I plan on making a move on 'one day'. So why not today?

If you have the question '*what would I like to learn this winter?*', it gives you a timeframe to aim for and sets your mind off on a search of what *would* light you up. You can go to external classes or perhaps commit a certain amount of time each week to self-study.

Something that comes to mind for me is completing the exercises in the book '*Style Statement: Live by Your Own Design*' by Danielle LaPorte and Carrie McCarthy. I borrowed this book from the library years ago and started going through all the questions. I did not finish it before the book was due back and never borrowed the book again or bought my own copy. The answers I have written so far are illuminating and I know I want to go back and finish the exercises in that book.

Another thing that I want to do is practice using my spinning wheel. When I was in my early teens, I learned to spin wool. I know, it does sound a bit '*Little House on the Prairie*' but I enjoyed it, plus I would knit the wool I spun. Unbelievably, my spinning wheel was still at my dad's house after thirty-plus years, so I reclaimed it (dad was thrilled to be rid of it) and now have it in my home ready to go.

Yes, my husband did give me 'the look' – you know the look that says 'when are you *ever* going to use that?' as my dusty old spinning wheel was being carried into our house. The look also said 'do I know you at all?' because he did not know I spun wool. I admit I have not used it yet, but I will. All I need are a few YouTube videos and a carded wool purchase (although I did learn to card my own wool too) and *an intention with a deadline.*

That last one is the most important thing which will help you achieve any goal.

I have just thought of something else for my project list too – I have always wanted to learn to sing. Just for myself, I don't want to perform; but I love singing out loud when it is only me around. I know it would help my breathing too (I seem to hold my breath and often must take deep breaths). To learn, I would probably have a look on YouTube first but I imagine I would need to take proper lessons from someone. At least doing a few YouTube videos will get me started.

These things would all make fantastic winter projects. Thinking about them and noting them down gets them out of my head and it is more likely I will act on them.

What might be on your wish-list if you searched all the corners of your mind?

Keep active

As cozy as it is to be at home on the sofa when it is cold and the fire is going, it does feel good to move around and *do* something. If it is not raining or too windy outside, I like to go for a walk soon after it is light in the morning. This way, I have gotten my exercise out of the way for the day, in case waning enthusiasm or rough weather closing in hampers me later.

When I am reluctant to go out for a walk, I tell myself it will be nice and cozy to rug up and get some air. It also feels good to be out amongst the world. Those thoughts combined with the prospect of an uplifting podcast, audiobook or my favourite music helps me feel happy about going out in the cold, and I return home bursting with motivation and new ideas to work on.

If I do not go for a walk first thing; just before or just after lunch is another good time. Sometimes it is nice to mix things up and not do the same routine every day. If the weather is looking threatening, even a short stroll around the neighbourhood is beneficial. I carry an umbrella and usually wear my rain-jacket too.

If the weather is truly 'indoors-only', I would like to say that I put an exercise DVD on, and I do have quite a few, but I do not ever watch them. I wish I could but they just do not appeal. When I put in a yoga DVD, I last about five minutes. While I have completed the whole workout from a fitness DVD once, I have never done it again.

I think I just much prefer to be outdoors and, if I am at home, would rather be productive with jobs. Why jump around on the spot in front of the television, when I could use that same time and energy to do the housework?

On days when I am at home, it feels good to do one sitting down activity and then one moving around activity (keeping warm is an added bonus). For example, I will write a blog post or reconcile my banking, then vacuum or hang the washing out. Have lunch watching a television programme then go out for a stroll around the neighbourhood. Do some hand-sewing then chop vegetables for dinner. Read a few chapters of my book then bring the washing in and fold it.

By doing this you get rest time, and you get jobs done.

If you wear a Fitbit or pedometer to count your steps, you will find all these movements add up.

Be social

I adore winter, where I can hibernate without having people think I am too much of a hermit, but even I realise that being social can feel good.

When it starts to feel like all I am doing is going to work, coming home, going to work and coming home; I know it is time to suggest to my husband that we expand our world for just an evening by inviting friends over or going out somewhere.

Something I have come back to after a long hiatus are board games. We hosted a family game night where we played *Cranium*, which was such a nice change. Just for fun, we moved the dining table into the middle of our living room and set up for the game to be the main attraction.

Another time we visited friends with small children, and after their kids were in bed we played *Uno* all night.

At first you might think '*games?*', and not be that keen because games do not sound as sexy as going out for dinner or seeing a movie at the theatre for example, but just give them a go. Others might not be keen at first either but once you are going, you will see that everyone is enjoying themselves and afterwards they will probably talk about that great night you all had.

And it means you can be social with others and not just sit there looking at each other, having food and drink be all there is to focus on. You still converse, chat and catch up with each other, but it adds another dimension to the conversation and, I find, brings everyone closer together.

I have not pieced a jigsaw together in a long time, but the thought appeals. That might be even less appealing than a games night for some though. I can imagine the invitees saying '*Fiona has just invited us around to do a jigsaw, do you think she has lost her mind?*' But perhaps if the jigsaw was there as part of the evening and not the main attraction, it would be okay. Or maybe I will just keep my jigsaw dream for myself.

I also like to be social during the day with my female friends. It is nice to meet for lunch or coffee and have a catch-up for an hour or two. It is especially nice if you have not seen each other in a while, to contact or be contacted for a get-together.

As an introvert, I am quite happy being social by myself too. Sometimes if I want to research clothing options for the upcoming season or need to do the banking, I will make a small outing of it. I will go into the city and have a stroll around by myself. I am not prone to impulse buys and will come home empty-handed mostly, having just enjoyed having a look around. This might not be the best suggestion for an outing if you have trouble not shopping. Or maybe you can go, but not take any of your cards, just enough cash for the bus or parking, and a hot drink.

Going one step further than any of the above suggestions, why not make up your guest room? You will then be ready for weekend or overnight guests. It is so nice not to feel panic-stricken when you receive a call that your cousin and his wife are coming to visit your city for a function and could they stay the night? Or if your friends with young children are over for dinner, you are more than happy to open the door to your neat and tidy guest room when the kids get tired.

Having the guest room organized, which I think ends up being the storage and junk room in most households, gives you much more spontaneity and you might even think to yourself *'who could we invite from out of town to stay for the weekend?'*

Chapter 4.
Work on feeling good

It is important to keep your vibration high at any time of the year, and especially so when it is cold. It can be easier to feel deflated in winter and let small things get on top of you. By actively focusing on keeping your frequency elevated, you will happily make better choices because you want to, not because you should do (which does not feel as good and does not provide lasting motivation).

How to feel good in the winter then? We have already talked about keeping healthy by moving your body daily (even if only for a short time), and having good, healthy food that fills you up and keeps you warm.

Next are *all the lovely things* – enjoying and feeling nurtured by your home; dressing in a way that pleases you, which is comfortable and cozy; and feeling inspired to keep your grooming up, which helps you feel presentable and on top of things.

Lastly, I have a few tips to help you feel better if you do have a period of mild flatness.

Home as your winter sanctuary

As gorgeous as it is in the summer months when you can leave the doors open and your house is warm all the time, there is great comfort in nesting in the winter. I love the layered look with a cozy throw rug on the sofa, inviting cushions and a candle flickering.

Cozy up your home by decluttering the living areas and adding comforting touches such as a candle in a pretty holder and a fluffy throw to snuggle up in. Declutter books and magazines and display a few new titles, much like a hotel would.

Give your living area a good cleaning; it will feel so much better and you will keep warm too. When I have a day at home, I often find it is cold in the morning, even after a hot shower. I want to sit down and read or write, but I do not want to switch on heating or light the fire because I know the sun will warm our house within a few hours.

This makes morning the perfect time for me to heat myself up by doing my housework. Once I have done the cleaning, I might inspire myself by viewing my current favourite Instagram account – Ralph Lauren Home. I love the way Ralph does traditional home looks, and browsing a few images always motivates me to move things around and 'stage' different areas such as our coffee or dining table, or switch cushion covers on the sofa.

I do not have a lot in the way of seasonal décor, but I do like to change things up occasionally to bring a visual freshness to my home. Small projects such as organising and dusting my bookshelves is a cozy way to spend a few hours, and my books look so much more appealing afterwards, especially if I have managed to declutter a few.

There are also things we have done to insulate our home to make it look and feel warmer. When we moved in, we took advantage of government subsidies to install under-floor insulation and a wood-burner.

At the same time, we also changed the old, dark navy curtains in our living room to inexpensive ready-made thermal calico curtains, adding sheer drapes both for privacy and to trap warmth in the winter. In the summer, they shade the room nicely and filter the light. I notice that a lot of fancy hotels have beautiful sheer curtains too.

If the weather is fine but cool, it is quite pleasant to spend an hour or so tidying up our garden – trimming the Buxus hedge (it is quite small, so I do it with hand-held hedge-clippers), weeding garden beds and maybe cutting a few flowers to put in bud-vases inside.

It is particularly satisfying to have done this and then be inside when it starts raining afterwards. The garden looks refreshed from my pottering and now it is being watered. Our yard is nothing fancy and I am not a great gardener, but to have it neatly kept brings me great pleasure when I look out the window.

After a busy and productive morning, I then have my lunch and enjoy relaxing time in the afternoon. I might go for a walk outside, sew, make dinner, read, or watch a movie and knit.

Dress in clothes that make you feel good

If you are going to enjoy the winter months, you'd better be dressed in clothes that make you feel good. In that perfect, shimmery mirage of a life (the perfect you), you would have a curated closet of items that make you feel fabulous and have people complimenting you at every turn.

The perfect you loves the texture of everything she wears – both to look at and the feeling against your skin – and you feel like a million dollars every morning. When you leave the house, you are not surprised when fashion bloggers stop you so they can take your photo.

Nah, that has never happened to me either, and if I can cobble together an outfit of a day, that's an achievement. Or it was before I started getting my act together. As winters passed by and I bemoaned my uninspiring wardrobe, I knew nothing would change if I did not do anything. I knew it was up to me to make my winter wardrobe something to look forward to wearing; a wardrobe I felt cozy and cosseted in and looked amazing in at the same time.

Something I now love to do at the beginning of a new season is to create my capsule wardrobe. This winter I did it 'officially' by joining Courtney Carver's Project 333

movement. When I say join, you do not actually 'join', you just do it. The idea is to create a capsule wardrobe of 33 pieces for the upcoming three months. You can read about it on Courtney's website here:
http://bemorewithless.com/project-333/

Courtney counts shoes and accessories in her 33, but I did not count shoes for mine. To keep it simple, I chose 33 items of clothing and a few accessories that all mix and match. I thought 33 would not be enough, but I only got up to 32 and I already had a few accessories to bulk up the numbers.

The most important thing is to create a winter wardrobe that excites you. Find your fashion uniform and build on that, then you can carry on with other things knowing you have stuff to wear for the current season. There are so many reasons to love having a capsule wardrobe:

Ease of getting ready in the morning

Feeling like you are all organised, not just getting dressed, but in life!

A roadmap for the season ahead – there are no

surprises

Seeing straight away if you have a full wardrobe for the season or if you need to fill in some gaps

Feeling like you are that chic and elegant woman who plans her wardrobe out

Having a colour-coordinated mix-and-match selection

Having checked that everything is comfortable and in good order so you can focus on other things instead of wardrobe mishaps

Being more creative in your choices and wearing some of your lovely pieces that you may pass over because they are 'too good/delicate/fancy'

Doing something like Project 333 helps you see where you have gaps in your wardrobe. When I was planning my winter capsule, I could see I had hardly any cozy long-sleeved tops. I took an afternoon to look around the shops and found a fine merino-knit cowl-neck top at *Farmers*, an inexpensive department store here in New

Zealand. It was just what I wanted, so I bought it in black.

After a few weeks, I realized how much I was loving it and how cozy the cowl was around my neck, so I went back and bought the other two colours it came in – teal and a soft red, both slightly melange in look. Pairing these with skinny or straight jeans and low-heeled suede ankle boots gave me a very useful base for my everyday wardrobe.

When you are going through your clothing for the upcoming season, be brave and declutter any clothing items you are not excited about seeing again. It is very tempting to keep something because you might like it again next year, especially if that item cost you a bit of money. I know because I have done this myself. I know from experience though, that if you do not want to wear it this winter, you are unlikely to want to wear it next winter. Give yourself a break from the guilt and put it into your donation box.

I read a great quote recently that said something along the lines of 'when you let something go it is a decision you make once, but when you keep something that is not really adding to your life, you have to make the decision to keep it over and over'. That spoke to me and I remember it when I know I need to get rid of something, yet a part of me is holding back.

I do not read a ton of fashion magazines and I would not consider fashion a great passion of mine (style yes, fashion no), but even I find it exciting to check out the new fashions and style forecasts for the season. I love to see the new colours coming through as well as old favourites.

Plum is a shade that I love to incorporate in autumn and winter. It feels very rich and cozy to me, and goes well with my colouring. With my 'soft summer' colouring I go for a muted and soft heathered plum rather than a crisp or jewel shade plum.

Dependent on your colouring, there will be those favoured shades that make you think of the upcoming winter season. Incorporate these into your wardrobe when you are putting together your winter pieces.

Texture and the feel of a fabric against your skin is very important too. When I analysed why I continued to avoid wearing certain items, even if I liked them hanging up, it was because I did not like the fabric against my skin. Maybe it was synthetic that felt slithery, or a wool top that was too scratchy. After I gave myself permission to be the diva with sensitive skin, it was an easy decision to declutter these items.

Summer can be too hot for scarves, but winter gives you a chance to accessorise around the neck. I love the current fashion for big chunky scarves; however, since I have been having a cowl-neck winter, I have not been wearing my winter scarves as much. In addition, I live in a sub-tropical area where we do not get truly cold winters, so scarves are often for looks rather than warmth. I may go back to scarves next year though.

That is good to remember too – just because you choose a minimalist capsule to dress in this season, does not mean you must limit yourself to those same clothes in the future. The fun of capsule dressing is that you are making up a collection for the season, much like a fashion designer would.

Then, in future seasons, you can choose to wear the same or a very similar capsule again, or you can change the direction either in colour or style. My outfits do not change radically from season to season because I keep my clothes for quite a long time. Even inexpensive clothes can last if you treat them well.

Another fun way to think about creating a capsule wardrobe if you are having trouble starting, is to think about it as if you were going away on a three-month long working holiday at your company's New York, London or Paris office (take your pick).

You probably could not pile your whole closet into a suitcase, so what would you take that would mix and match, make you feel comfortable and happy and look good? If you had two suitcases open on your bed and you could only take clothes, shoes and accessories that would fit into those suitcases, what would you pack? It is quite a fun exercise.

I did something similar last year, but for real, when my husband and I had a four-night Sydney mini-break. We decided to take carry-on luggage only, so I practiced a week before just how I was going to pack my tiny Samsonite carry-on bag. And I did it! What a proud moment and it showed me how a little prior planning meant I could dress happily in a capsule wardrobe on our trip. The post detailing this is on my blog here: http://www.howtobechic.com/2016/05/the-chic-travel-wardrobe.html

If you have never tried a capsule wardrobe before, why not have a play with one right now? It does not matter if you are in the middle of a season, you can still look at what you have, see what your favourite outfits are, lay all the hangers out on your bed and start counting your items. Everything that is not going into your own personal fashion collection for the season can be put aside for now.

If it is the middle of the season, this is almost a better time to start as a beginner; because you have already had some experience with your clothes for that season, and you can see what you are enjoying wearing, and what you are bypassing. Move the clothes you are not wearing – without guilt – to another closet and see what gaps you have that you could browse the mid-season sales for.

These days it seems there are beginning-of-season-sales, mid-season-sales and end-of-season-sales, so you will probably never need to pay full price for anything. My three merino cowl tops that I wore a lot this winter were new stock half-price at the beginning of the season. Total score.

One last thing to mention which I think is an important part of your capsule wardrobe is *perfume*. I love perfume so much that I often get more excited about what perfume I am going to wear that day than what outfit – I know, it sounds silly but I do!

Entirely selfishly, I wear perfumes to please myself. I am no longer a perfume snob and enjoy both high-end and low-end fragrances. Some days I am in the mood for light and playful, while other days I prefer to feel sophisticated and elegant. It can be comforting to spritz on a warm enveloping perfume to complete your cozy 'look' for the day.

For me, fragrance starts as soon as I get out of the shower – perhaps I will apply a rich, vanilla-scented body cream to my arms and décolletage, then layer on one of my current winter scents such as Givenchy Organza.

If you love smelling nice, wear your favourite cool-weather perfumes every day and look out for delicious body products you can layer them with. *Bath and Body Works* and *Victoria's Secret* have body creams and lotions that smell divine and at reasonable prices.

If you want to research new fragrances, check out my favourite perfume website Fragrantica (http://www.fragrantica.com/). It is a wonderful resource which has helped me identify notes that I love and those that I don't. Type in your favourite perfume and see what genre it belongs to. I love to find out inexpensive dupes for my favourites too; it is all there.

Be cozy when you are at home

I may have mentioned this before (once or twice or fifty times), but I love being at home. It's an introvert's favourite place to be. As well as making home welcoming and cozy, I love to feel comforted by the clothes I choose to wear at home. I enjoy changing into my lounge wear as soon as I get home, but I also want to feel productive, and not like a slouch in pyjamas.

It pays to take some time and even invest a small amount of money into clothes specifically for home to keep you warm and have you feeling comfortable. It is hard to get motivated to do something if your ankles are cold or the top you are wearing is constrictive.

In the winter, I like to buy a couple of new pairs of leggings exclusively for home wear. Last year I had navy and black cotton knit leggings, but this year I paid a tiny bit more and went for slinkier viscose knit leggings – two pairs in black, so I always have a new pair when the other is in the wash. I also bought one matching black top plus I have another couple of knit tops that I wear with them at home.

This outfit falls between pyjamas, and clothes that I wear out in public. I would never wear my lounge clothes out, but if someone comes to the door I don't look like I've just rolled out of bed. I always style my hair – often in a bun or ponytail, and I wear soft slip-on shoes like *Skechers Go Walks*, or my short black sheepskin *Ugg* boots if it is colder.

I always imagine myself in the future (that perfect future where my life is perfect and I am perfect too) wearing the same outfits at home as I do to go to work or out, but I just love to feel comfortable and free to move when I am at home. Sitting down writing at my desk is more comfortable in leggings than jeans, and when I am doing my housework, it is much easier to bend or kneel when I am in my stretchy outfits.

I have learned to declutter the guilt that is associated with what I think I 'should' be wearing. There is no point in guilt, and it is only me putting pressure on myself, no-one else; so, now I wear my lounge wear with pleasure.

In the evening when I have finished my jobs and we are relaxing after dinner, I change my shoes for a big pair of fluffy socks (in my mind this is my 'supermodel relaxing by the log fire in Aspen' look; I highly doubt the reality is so). Often I will put a rich moisturiser on my feet and put my socks back on, and it is so relaxing to curl up on the sofa with a book, movie or television programme, a cat near me and my husband next to me.

Have a think about what you would love to wear at home that would make you feel relaxed, comfortable, productive and organized. You want a few outfits that are attractive, easy to wear and, if you are like me, not too expensive.

You might not choose all-black like my current outfits (my husband called these my 'cat burglar' clothes when I first wore them); rather you might like to wear brighter or more feminine colours than you typically wear outside the home. That is a goal of mine for the forthcoming season; to find a couple of home lounge wear outfits that are exactly that – elegant and sensual in flattering and elegant colours.

One of the characters at the beginning of the movie *Sideways* wore pale pink satin drawstring pants with a lacy sleeveless top and little scuffs at home. My husband commented when we were watching this movie that it would be a nice home outfit for me because he knows I like to wear silky and fine fabrics that are feminine and attractive, and I like to be comfortable too.

The bonus of wearing lounge wear that makes you feel fabulous is that you are more likely to eat better, and not snack on junk food all afternoon because of dressing in scruffy slob-about clothes.

Take care of your grooming

'*How you do one thing is how you do everything*'. I love this quote so much and often remind myself of it for the inspiration it provides when I am tempted to be a slob.

An example of this is with my grooming. Ever since I made the decision to moisturise my body daily, no matter what, it has had a positive effect on other areas of my life. Even in the winter when it is quite cold when I get out of the shower and I would rather throw my clothes on straight away, I still do it. I have been moisturising daily for so long now that it has become a habit, much like brushing my teeth.

I am sure the condition of my skin has improved too – taking care of yourself comes from the inside out and the outside in. So, by eating healthy food and drinking water as well as hydrating from the outside, your skin will look better than if you did either or neither.

It can be hard to keep your grooming up in the winter, but by choosing one thing to do religiously, you will find it easier to keep up other areas as well. Say you choose to shave your legs two or three times a week despite no-one else seeing them (except for you and your man of course, only the two most important people in your life).

Even if you make once a week your absolute minimum, it is still better than neglecting your legs the whole winter. You will feel better about yourself, more feminine and like the glamorous woman you know you are deep down.

After going back to shaving my legs from waxing, I am now having my legs waxed again. I am monitoring whether I think the money spent is worth the ease, and at this moment ease is winning. It is nice to not have to think about shaving my legs, and I use that time to exfoliate with scratchy gloves and shower gel instead. Doing this then putting on body lotion afterwards feels so good.

Another area I love to look after are my feet, in particular my heels. My biggest horror is to have thick, cracked dry heels and so I often use my scratchy shower gloves on my feet, as well as applying shea butter body cream before putting on my fluffy home socks.

On a friend's recommendation, I bought myself an inexpensive little gadget called an *Emjoi Micro-Pedi Callus Remover*. It spins around like a tiny sander and my goodness, it is fantastic. Make sure to put a towel under your feet while you're using it because of the white dust that is produced, but it is so quick and easy to give your heels a quick 'sand' each week.

You will feel pampered by your own self-care doing this and your heels will emerge for summer as if you have just returned from a European spa. I like to give my toenails a break from colour in the winter, and then when summer comes it is fun to paint them in a bright or dark crème colour. In saying that, sometimes I like to do the complete opposite and paint my toenails in the middle of winter for a few weeks. Doing something out of your normal regime can lift your spirits I find.

It is the same with my fingernails. Mostly I keep them short and unpolished, however sometimes it is enjoyable to paint them, even though I know they will chip within a week or two. After all, I put makeup on knowing I am going to wash it off at the end of the day, why not have a little fun with my nails as well.

The more pampering you do for yourself, the better you feel and the more you will do. It has a flow-on and expanding effect.

The opposite occurs also – the less you do, the more slobby and unmotivated you feel; so, enjoy your femininity and indulge in all the little things from time to time. It is not decadent; it is *necessary* to your wellbeing.

Keep well

I am generally a very healthy person, and am grateful I have not had anything serious to deal with, but even I sometimes find it a struggle in the winter. I have never had proper depression, but from time to time, right back to my teens I have had the occasional bout of mild melancholia.

Normally I love the coziness of winter but sometimes I can feel flat. I need to remember that winter is naturally a time for us to slow down and take better care of ourselves. I also need to remember that eating rubbish food makes you feel rubbish. You are guaranteed the same result every time!

All of us are a work in progress, and some of us need the contrast that comes with not taking care of ourselves to show us what we would rather experience. It feels good to honour our health and nurture ourselves with good food, rest and plenty of hydration.

It is sometimes easier to treat yourself as if you were looking after someone else; it certainly is for me. I might not make myself a proper lunch and instead nibble on unhealthy processed carbs, yet when I make lunch for someone else, I make sure it is an appealing and nutritionally balanced meal.

Therefore, it can be a helpful idea to put together a lunch plate as if you were making it for a guest. Preparing a meal from this angle helps with motivation to include the finishing touches such as fresh chopped herbs that you might skip if it was 'just you'. Interesting, don't you think?

Drinking water is especially important in the summer when it is hot, however hydration is still vital in the cold months. Our health is created from the inside out, so keeping fluids flowing into your body will help with dry skin, for example. When you need to warm up, it is nice to have a mug of hot water near you to sip from, or an herbal tea such as peppermint, ginger or the many varieties of fruit teas that are available.

To assist my health, at the beginning of winter I make sure to buy a new container of fish oil and I take one capsule each morning. It means I do not have to feel so bad about not eating as much fish in the winter and the oil will make my eyes, hair and skin healthy.

The only other supplement I stock up on is

1000mg vitamin C tablets, which I take if I feel a sniffle coming on. I learned years ago that you can stave off a cold by taking 10,000mg of vitamin C each day until you feel better. If you already have a cold, you can shorten it by doing the same thing.

I count out ten tablets and take one each hour until they are all gone for the day. It works for me every time. This winter I felt a tickle in my nose on a Monday, come Tuesday I had a full-blown head cold. I started taking my vitamin C 'cure' straight away and I was much better by Thursday. Four days! I hear people talk about having winter lurgies for weeks. No thank you.

To avoid bugs in the first place, be extra vigilant about washing your hands in the winter (and keep a lightweight handcream nearby to prevent your hands from chapping).

Chapter 5.

Keep your motivation up

As winter wears on you may find yourself becoming tired. It is easier to be irritated and you might find yourself forgetting things. It is at times like this when you can find everyday life overwhelming and not feeling like your usual self.

You have probably felt like this before and emerged fine, but it is not nice to feel out of sorts. Accepting that it is only a phase and making plans to help yourself feels better though. Logically you know that more early nights, less computer time and more good foods (especially protein) will help get you back into balance, but still, the opposites beckon.

If you feel like your tank is running on empty, and normal everyday interactions and problems are getting on top of you, try to simplify your life, at least for the next little while.

Everything in nature goes in cycles, and you might be in a strange one right now, but see this as a good thing. It helps you to know what you want and how you need to treat yourself.

Try these for starters:

Wonderfully early nights to bed. Instead of staying up until your normal bedtime out of habit, even though you might be flagging, start getting ready for bed one or even two hours earlier than usual. You will probably find you drop off to sleep easily.

Stay away from junky foods, especially sugar (which you crave more when feeling flat I have found) and make sure to include good, natural protein at each meal.

Limit screen-time after dinner. For me, this means I have the laptop shut down before we start dinner and watch one television programme.

Limit caffeine drinks and do not have any caffeine after mid-afternoon if you are sensitive to it.

Walk outside as many days as you can, even if it is just for a short stroll. Sunlight going into your pineal gland via your eyes is beneficial (do not wear sunglasses).

Do not leave too long between meals. Sometimes if I am busy at work, it could be 2-3pm before I eat lunch. Considering I had breakfast at about 8am and a soy latte mid-morning, that is too late. I need to be more organised with having lunch ready to go, rather than get to 1pm and start preparing it (and be ready for the inevitable interruptions that goes along with working in retail).

Tidy up your surroundings. Because it is coming into the new season now, we have many deliveries at our retail business. This means unpacking, pricing and photographing for my husband, and 'cutting out' the photos then loading onto the website for me. We also both work in our store in addition to doing all the administration and everything else that comes with running your own business.

I am sure you are similarly busy at home and/or work. This means less urgent work can be pushed to the background, such as filing, tidying and organizing. But those things when left undone contribute to stress, so focus on doing the important as well as the urgent jobs.

Completing small tasks. Don't you find it is the little things, unfinished, that bother you the most? As you go through your day, try to complete small tasks as you come across them, and enjoy the boost in energy when you do so.

Be around nice people. Keeping away from people that get you down is important because they affect you more when you are feeling tired. Worry and stress do not help you feel better.

It is not always possible of course (I deal with many different types of people at work and I am sure you do too), but I have realised that dealing with horrid people who will be unhappy no matter what, can be minimized. It helps me to see it is their problem not mine, and I can limit or eliminate my time with them. Life is just too short to be around nasty people.

Be gentle with yourself, and do not do too much if you do not want to. Rather than a whirlwind marathon housework day, just do the basics and spend some time relaxing and reading (no guilt allowed).

Remember to breathe. You may find yourself holding onto your breath. It feels such a relief to let it flow in... and out. Remind yourself as often as you need to – it could be many times a day. It certainly is for me.

Talk to someone. Let your other half know if you are feeling lower than normal and that you might need some TLC. The few times I have told my husband I was feeling low, not only did I feel better having shared it, but he had some helpful suggestions and looked out for me as well.

Clear out clutter corners at home and work. If an area is bothering you, even if you have other things to do, sort out that clutter corner. It often only takes a small amount of time, and you feel infinitely better and more able to tackle the harder jobs instantly.

Say no. No to library books that do not hold your attention, no to television programmes or movies you have recorded and decided you do not like, no to requests from others that you do not want to do. It can feel hard and like you are letting people down, but learning to say no is so beneficial to your mental health.

If you get a niggling feeling in your stomach when you think about something, decide there and then to do something about it (rather than putting it off). A weight is lifted immediately and you realise how things like this can weigh heavily on you.

Indulge in the little luxuries. Use all your lovely things and do not feel guilty at all. Spray on Chanel to go for a walk. Wear your pearl earrings to do the housework. Write in the brand-new journal you received as a gift. Buy yourself the richest dark chocolate you can find and enjoy a piece.

You may find it does not take much to turn things around, so that you feel sunnier again. Often you only need a good night's sleep because things always look better in the morning.

I love to open one of my favourite French Chic genre books to gain a little inspiration too – perhaps Anne Barone or Jennifer L. Scott. Borrow someone else's enthusiasm to give you a lift, so you can pump up your own again. Or, write your own inspiration in your journal. Ask yourself *'what would I like to hear right now?'*

Do things quickly

When it is cold, I am always tempted to stay in bed a little longer and put off getting into the shower because I am so warm and snuggly, but this just makes getting up worse.

Now I make it a game to do something as quickly as possible and then I have no option but to GO! If I ask myself *'how quickly can I do this job'*, I get it done so fast and then I have more time to do other things that I want to do. When I procrastinate and muck around 'because it's cold', I don't get nearly as much done and it feels horrible.

Say if I have a to-do list with seven items on it; what I used to do was resent that list and work through it at a snail's pace, doing other more fun things in between jobs. The result is that I would get through to the end of the day having not completed everything 'because I ran out of time' (I would moan to my poor husband), *and* I would have no down-time either.

My 'new' technique of doing things quickly works much better, as you would imagine. You can expand time to accommodate anything you like this way – I promise! Just the simple act of asking '*how quickly can I do this?*' changes the way your mind works and you will become effortlessly motivated to whizz through your list.

You may have heard that a job expands to fill the time available. That is true as well. If you have one week to complete a project, it will take one week. When I had a deadline of Father's Day to complete a gift idea I planned to make my dad, yes, you're correct, I finished the gift the night before.

What if you took your one-week project and gave yourself one day to finish it? I bet you could, and with not too much discomfort either. Doing this focuses your mind. You only need to try this once to prove it to yourself.

By the same token, take today's to-do list and give yourself half a day to complete all the tasks. Some might only take ten minutes to do, and the thought of doing them might have been more painful than the actual doing (this happens *all the time* to me).

You might think the suggestion to '*do things quickly*' will wear you out, but I have found the opposite – I become more efficient and have more energy afterwards. How crazy is that?

If you are a summer person

I have friends and family members who are summer people. They can become down in the winter season and only perk up if they are able to take a holiday somewhere hot. They bask happily in temperatures that I would find uncomfortable. What to do if you are one of those hot-weather people? Or perhaps you do not mind winter, but need a little bit of a sunshine break?

Here are a few ideas:

Can you move? This is not as silly as it sounds. If you really do dislike the winters where you live, can you move somewhere warmer? What is stopping you? Sometimes we live where we live, just because we live there.

I used to reside in Christchurch, in the colder South Island of New Zealand. It was a beautiful city and I loved the history and natural beauty, but gosh it was chilly, even in the summer. My cousin, who still lives there, used to joke that you could see the sun but not feel it.

I now live in Auckland, much further north and it is balmy by comparison. I have not worn a big winter coat since 1998 when I left

Christchurch.

I talk a lot about Brian Tracy's zero-based thinking, but that's because it works. It strips out everything else around a possible decision and helps you look at possibilities. Ask yourself *'knowing what we now know, if we could start all over again and choose where we wanted to live, would it be here? If not here, then where?'*

If your answer is 'somewhere else', consider your options. Investigate the job market, research schooling, ask your company whether you can work virtually or if there is another office you can transfer to.

This is unlikely to be a quick solution, but it is completely realistic. My husband and I started this exact process eighteen months ago and decided to move from the city we live in to a tiny town more than 400km (250 miles) away. The wheels are in motion now – we will have moved within six months and are both so excited about our 'new life'.

If you like where you live or cannot move right now, how can you conjure up summer in other ways?

Get some sun. Go out daily for a walk and a dose of Vitamin D. Rug up warm and wear your biggest movie-star sunglasses.

Book or plan a trip. Maybe you cannot go on a mid-winter vacation every year, but what about every second or third year? Planning and looking forward to a trip brings you almost as much pleasure as the trip itself – I have always believed this, and then I read there was a study proving it, so it must be true.

Decorate your home with summery touches. Maybe winter décor does not excite you; seeing all those throw rugs and coziness might depress you instead. So, why not decorate in a beachy theme as if it was the middle of summer? Have light-coloured linens and slip-covers, spring silk flowers, a beachy theme with blue-and-white ticking stripes, shell displays and candles set in sand inside hurricane lamps.

There is no law that says you must decorate for the season – go by your own rules and make it twelve months of summer at your house.

Watch summer movies and television programmes. You will no doubt have some favourite movies set in summer and/or warm climates; put those out for viewing during the winter. I know you may be thinking *'that's a* *lame idea, Fiona*' but I find that watching summer movies makes me feel happy and relaxed. Our mind does not know the difference between truth and lies, so if we choose to feel good by watching a summery movie, where's the harm in that?

One film that comes to mind for me is Woody Allen's *Vicky Cristina Barcelona*. It is set in Spain, and the air seems to shimmer with golden light and balmy heat. It is a real tonic to watch this movie on a cold winter's night. *To Catch a Thief* with Cary Grant and Grace Kelly is another wonderful movie that feels so summery and relaxing – you will feel inspired to be a more elegant person after watching this movie too.

Eat summery food. Sweetcorn might not be in season, but why not have an indoor barbeque anyway? You can cook steak and burgers on the stovetop, bake potatoes or make oven fries, and mix up some coleslaw. I cook my burger patties in the oven on a tray lined with baking paper and they brown nicely on both sides without the bother of getting out a frying pan.

A meal like this is just as filling and warming as a traditional winter meal and it can bring about the feeling of summer, as well as breaking up the long stretch of casseroles and oven bakes. And, I am sure you can get frozen corn-on-the-cob at the supermarket.

Wear tropical colours. Instead of dark winter colours, feel brighter by dressing in more summery shades. There are some gorgeous tropical colours which can be soft or bright. Coral and turquoise pair well with other shades for winter – think camel or coffee with turquoise, or coral with charcoal. Denim with white and navy always looks crisp and will not be out of place even in winter.

You could paint your finger- and toe-nails in a tropical hue, put on some sheer tangerine or mango-coloured lip gloss and dust bronzing powder (non-sparkly) where the sun would naturally touch your face – the tip of your nose, lightly across your forehead, and in a figure-3 down each side of your face – forehead, temple, cheekbone, jawline. I sometimes even put self-tanner on my décolletage and forearms in the middle of winter, just for a change.

Read a summer-issue magazine. Gather up some summer issues of your favourite magazines if you keep them, and have a flick through with your feet up. The only magazine I keep is the beautiful *Victoria*, and I find it so soothing to leaf through an issue. You may have home décor or cooking magazines that can bring a summery feel to your day, even if it is snowing outside.

Brighten up your light bulbs. A dull room in winter is not that enticing. I find it makes a huge difference if I have brighter light bulbs in lamps I want to read with, in the kitchen to work by and in my home office. If it is a dark day, I keep the lights on in daylight hours too; it just feels better.

There are special light bulbs you can get to help with the winter blues – they are called 'full spectrum' light bulbs.

Wear warm weather fragrances. I do love my rich and sweet winter fragrances, but every so often I will wear a perfume that is completely the opposite season. Fruity, citrus, aquatic or coconut – it feels like a tonic to wear a full-blown summery perfume in the middle of winter. Scent can change your mood in an instant, so why not wear something to feel brighter for the day?

Play light-hearted music. Rat Pack music always makes me think of summer. Make your own summer playlist to put on anytime you need a dose of sunshine and sand.

You might think these ideas won't do much, but just try one – they do! Changing your thinking state changes how you feel. You can do this internally by intentionally choosing the thoughts you think – changing a negative thought into its positive opposite to override the negative, and externally by the things you do. Give yourself the best chance of success and do both at once.

Make plans for the next six to twelve months

To me, a successful life is comprised of being happy and content in the present at the same time as looking forward to an exciting future. Having one or two things to look forward to – and they don't have to be big at all – helps keep your motivation up and your momentum going.

They could be family gatherings; dinner at a friend's house; having people stay with you; visiting a craft fair; anything. If you have nothing coming up, look at your calendar and see if there is something you can book in.

Plan little treats. My husband and I love to stay at our favourite five-star luxury hotel right here in the city where we live – just for the night. They always have good package deals and it's a mini-break we can have while running our seven-days-a-week business. We go for a hot swim in the roof-top pool, dress up for dinner, and generally live the glamorous life for twenty-four-hours, complete with white fluffy robes and a late checkout.

Daydream about the future. I do this myself by writing down lists of my ideal lifestyle, home, personal style and what kind of person I want to be; and with my husband talking about our dream home we'd love to have, and what we would do with tons of money if we won the lottery (not that we buy tickets, but still, it's fun).

Doing this is an excellent antidote to an uninspiring day, and we also come up with great ideas for the future. Something grandiose on our list, such as touring a French wine region, can become part of our plans soon (touring a wine region right near us on our summer holiday).

Think about your summer plans. While it can feel like winter is dragging on at times, the truth is that spring will be here in a few short months. It always feels like a small miracle when the spring weather arrives, even though you know it will – it always does.

I am not a big gardener, but I do get excited about planting a few terracotta pots with brightly coloured annuals such as petunias, impatiens and lobelia. I look forward to watering them each day and imagine the ebullient display they will provide.

Look at any upcoming birthdays, weddings or other special occasions. Plan so that you are not scrambling around at the last minute for a suitable gift or nice outfit to wear. You might even tack on a small holiday to an out-of-town wedding by taking a couple of extra days leave from work.

Planning ahead feels good because you are organised, plus you get extra time to look forward to the event.

Chapter 6.

Create your ideal chic winter season

Anything we experience, either good or bad, is because we choose to experience it that way. A lot changed for me when I fully understood that things do not just happen to us – we are in charge.

Why not choose for yourself how you want to experience your winter months and make those things happen that you would love to do. Don't just float along expecting everything to fall into place perfectly, because it probably will not.

I am guilty of this – I don't make choices and

then feel bad when I don't have a good time. Of course, we all need to go to work, drop the children at school and run our household, but we can still enjoy ourselves whilst doing these things, whether it's summer or winter.

Choose that you are going to have your most fun winter ever and you will. *Ask* yourself how you can have your best winter yet and you will come up with loads of ideas. Act as if you *love* winter, and all that comes with it, and you will find your mood does not drop with the barometer. Mind over matter!

Realise that your surroundings do not dictate how you feel; *you* dictate how you feel and ultimately what your surroundings will look like. Do not be led around like a horse on a lead – choose for yourself.

Bonus journal questions

To get you started, you will find in this chapter some of my favourite journaling questions to help you create the ideal chic winter of your dreams. Start at the beginning and go through this list sequentially, or choose the question that you find most appealing or easy. Write down 3-5 answers for each question, or free-flow and let yourself continue writing or typing.

If you think you won't get around to doing this, write out these journal questions – and any of your own that come to mind – in the back of a small notebook and have it with you. Then, when you are on your lunch break, waiting for an appointment or having a coffee outing for one, pull out your notebook and choose a question to start brainstorming ideas to.

I have a notebook like this and I have found so many great ideas from doing these exercises, plus, when I read back through it I feel supremely inspired. It feels like all the goodness is custom-made for my desires, tastes and happiness... because it is!

Do not let any doom and gloom into this notebook. If you must vent and get stuff out, have a separate notebook.

When I found myself divorced at thirty, I filled a hardcover notebook with my despair. Years later when I was organising, I came across it and realised there was nothing to be gained by keeping this journal. It had served its purpose, which was to be a repository for my turmoil and to work out my feelings. Thankfully, I was now out the other side and happier than ever, so I let it go (into the rubbish bin!)

Have fun with these journal questions and *inspire yourself.* Find out what you really want to experience this winter, and guide yourself through a gorgeous winter season laced with your own 'flavour'.

Let's choose one and get started!

1. What would be your ideal 'fantasy' winter experience this year? Write a paragraph or 5-10 bullet points.

2. Does your fantasy winter match your past 'reality' winters?

3. How can you bring your fantasy winter and your reality winter together?

4. What are your main goals this winter?

5. How can you look forward to winter?

6. What has gone well for you in past winters that you would like to include this winter?

7. What has not had such great results for you in past winters that you would like to avoid?

8. Taking your answers in the above question, change them into the opposite and write down five ways you can create this for each point you mention.

9. List 5-10 ways you can be more prepared this winter.

10. Start a winter menu plan for each of the three meals a day. Note down any favourites and see if you can make them healthier.

11. List five healthy snack options to have on hand.

12. What project(s) would you love to complete this winter?

13. What trip(s), long or short, would you love to take this winter?

14. If you took a staycation in your own town, what activities or day trips could you do?

15. If you had time off at home, what home project(s) would you love to complete?

16. Looking at your living area and master bedroom, brainstorm ideas to make these two areas a cozy sanctuary for winter.

17. Bring out all winter clothes from your closet and do a quick sort-through. You don't have to get rid of anything right now, but put aside anything that makes you feel frumpy, doesn't fit, or you don't like the texture or colour as much as other items etc.

18. Think of three words you would like to embody in your personal clothing style this

winter. For me, this past winter I chose *casual*, *cozy* and *chic*.

19. Put back in your closet only the items that reflect your winter essence words.

20. Consider storing away (or donating if you are sure) the other clothes and focus on your ideal wardrobe already hanging up.

21. Put together outfits (bonus points for taking photos, I like to lay mine out on the floor complete with shoes and accessories, as shown here:

    http://www.howtobechic.com/2016/05/the-seasonal-wardrobe-autumnspring.html)

22. If you like to change into lounge wear when you arrive home, do you have two or three comfortable and stylish outfits to wear? Research a few if you don't.

23. List 5-10 personal grooming upgrades you would do if time and money were no object. Look at that list and see how many you can include in your life starting this week.

24. Look at what supplements you might need and what practices you could put into place to keep good health this winter.

25. List all the little things that drain your energy the most, and brainstorm ways to improve or eliminate them from your life.

26. What are 5-10 ways you could bring summer into your life when it is cold and grey outside?

27. What do you have coming up to look forward to over the next 6-12 months?

28. What can you book into your calendar to look forward to over the next 6-12 months?

To finish

How much you get out of a season – and life – is entirely in your hands, entirely. No matter your personal situation, you can *always* make it feel better by the way you think about it.

If you think your life is humdrum and unexciting, I am sure there are ladies around the world who would love to have your life. It would be their *dream*. Think about all the wonderful people around you, and all the ways in which you are so, so lucky already.

Then, think of how you can make it *even better*. You deserve to experience a wonderful and fulfilling winter – the winter of your dreams – just because you are you.

This is something I am very passionate about because I have done a lot of work on it over the past couple of years, and the main thing to remember is that YOU ARE ENOUGH. If you are standing here, alive on this earth, you are enough and you are worth receiving everything your heart desires.

Think big and know that anything you can dream of is available to you.

I am still expanding what I know I am capable of and what I can achieve; it is an ongoing process, which is scary and thrilling all at the same time.

I wish you nothing but the best and I sincerely hope you've have found loads in this book to inspire you to enjoy your most fun and happy winter yet. Let the goodness flow on as you go through the seasons and create your best life – you only experience it once! The saying 'life is not a dress rehearsal' is not only a cliché, it is entirely true as well.

Go forth and enjoy yourself – you are a beautiful and capable person who can bring light to herself and everyone around her.

With all my best,
Fiona

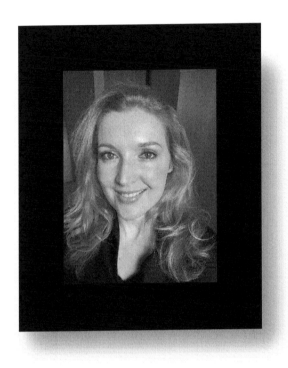

About the author

Fiona Ferris is passionate about, and has studied the topic of living well for more than twenty years, in particular that a simple and beautiful life can be achieved without spending a lot of money.

Fiona finds inspiration from all over the place including Paris and France, the countryside, big cities, fancy hotels, music, beautiful scents, magazines, books, all those fabulous blogs out there, people, pets, nature, other countries and cultures; really everywhere she looks.

Fiona lives in beautiful Auckland, New Zealand, with her husband, Paul, and their two rescue cats Jessica and Nina.

To learn more about Fiona, you can connect with her at:

howtobechic.com
fionaferris.com
facebook.com/fionaferrisauthor
twitter.com/fiona_ferris
instagram.com/fionaferrisnz
youtube.com/fionaferris

Fiona's other books, all available on Amazon:

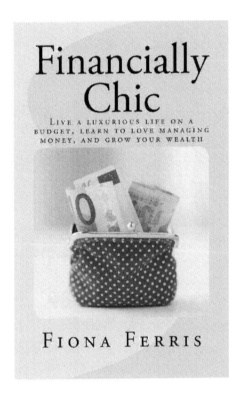

Financially Chic: Live a luxurious life on a budget, learn to love managing money, and grow your wealth

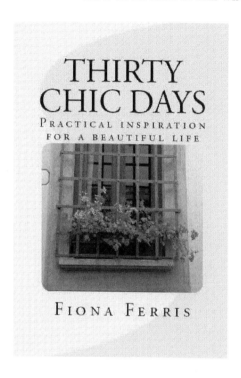

Thirty Chic Days: Practical inspiration for a beautiful life

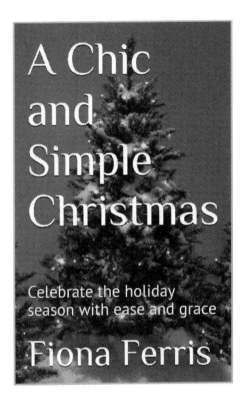

A Chic and Simple Christmas: Celebrate the holiday season with ease and grace

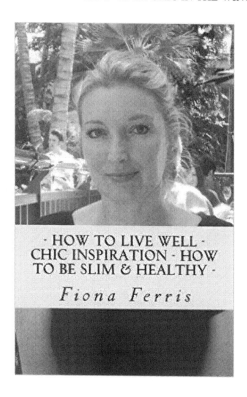

How to Live Well - Chic Inspiration - How to be Slim and Healthy (3-in-1 book)

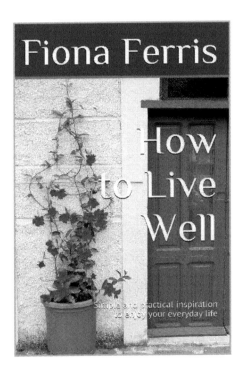

*How to Live Well: Simple and practical
inspiration to enjoy your everyday life*

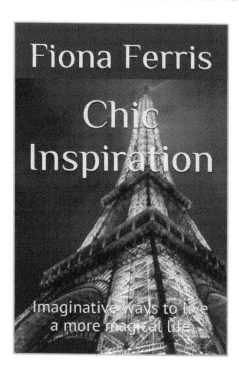

Chic Inspiration: Imaginative ways to live a more magical life

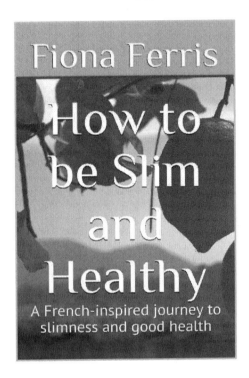

How to be Slim and Healthy: A French-inspired journey to slimness and good health

Printed in Great Britain
by Amazon